[DK] American College of Physicians

HOME MEDICAL GUIDE *to*

THYROID PROBLEMS

American College of Physicians

HOME MEDICAL GUIDE *to*

THYROID PROBLEMS

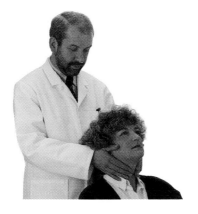

MEDICAL EDITOR
DAVID R. GOLDMANN, MD

ASSOCIATE MEDICAL EDITOR
DAVID A. HOROWITZ, MD

A DORLING KINDERSLEY BOOK

IMPORTANT

The American College of Physicians (ACP) Home Medical Guides provide general information on a wide range of health and medical topics. These books are not substitutes for medical diagnosis, and you should always consult your doctor on personal health matters before undertaking any program of therapy or treatment. Various medical organizations have different guidelines for diagnosis and treatment of the same conditions; the American College of Physicians–American Society of Internal Medicine (ACP–ASIM) has tried to present a reasonable consensus of these opinions.

Material in this book was reviewed by the ACP–ASIM for general medical accuracy and applicability in the United States; however, the information provided herein does not necessarily reflect the specific recommendations or opinions of the ACP–ASIM. The naming of any organization, product, or alternative therapy in these books is not an ACP–ASIM endorsement, and the omission of any such name does not indicate ACP–ASIM disapproval.

DORLING KINDERSLEY
LONDON, NEW YORK, AUCKLAND, DELHI,
JOHANNESBURG, MUNICH, PARIS, AND SYDNEY

DK www.dk.com

Senior Editors Jill Hamilton, Nicki Lampon
Senior Designer Jan English
DTP Design Jason Little
Editor Nicholas Mulcahy
Medical Consultant Anthony Jennings, MD

Senior Managing Editor Martyn Page
Senior Managing Art Editor Bryn Walls

Published in the United States in 2000 by
Dorling Kindersley Publishing, Inc.
95 Madison Avenue, New York, New York 10016

2 4 6 8 10 9 7 5 3 1

Library of Congress Catalog Card Number 99-76860
ISBN 0-7894-4173-X

Reproduced by Colourscan, Singapore
Printed and bound in the United States by Quebecor World, Taunton, Massachusetts

Contents

Introduction

The thyroid gland lies in the front of the neck between the skin and the voice box. The gland has a right and a left lobe, each about two inches in length. The entire thyroid gland weighs less than an ounce.

Despite its small size, the thyroid gland is an extremely important organ that controls our metabolism and is responsible for the normal functioning of every cell in the body. The thyroid achieves this by manufacturing the hormones known as thyroxine (T4) and triiodothyronine (T3) and by secreting these hormones into the bloodstream.

Iodine is an important constituent of these hormones. There are four atoms of iodine in each molecule of thyroxine, hence the abbreviation T4, and three atoms of iodine in each molecule of triiodothyronine or T3. Doctors believe that T4 only starts to be active when it is converted, mainly in the liver, to T3 by the removal of one atom of iodine.

In parts of the world with a severe lack of iodine in the diet, such as the Himalayas, there is not enough iodine for the thyroid gland to make adequate amounts of T3 and T4. In an attempt to compensate, the thyroid gland

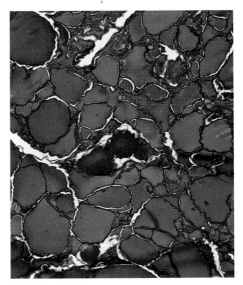

INSIDE THE THYROID
This microscope picture of the thyroid gland shows the thyroid follicles (seen here as blue), collections of cells that produce thyroid hormones. The orange patches are areas of stored hormones.

Location of the Thyroid Gland

This diagram shows the position of the thyroid within the neck. It is a butterfly-shaped gland consisting of two lobes in the lower neck, one on each side of the trachea, or windpipe, joined by a connecting layer of thyroid tissue.

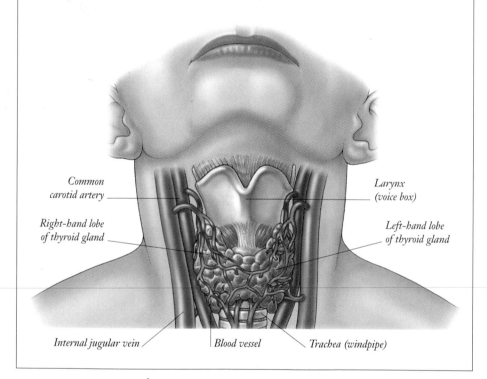

Common carotid artery

Right-hand lobe of thyroid gland

Larynx (voice box)

Left-hand lobe of thyroid gland

Internal jugular vein

Blood vessel

Trachea (windpipe)

enlarges enough to become visible and is then known as a goiter. If this extra manufacturing capacity is still inadequate, the patient develops an underactive thyroid gland (see p.30). Iodine deficiency is not present in the US. In some cases, too much iodine in the diet causes the thyroid gland to produce excessive amounts of thyroid hormones. This can also be a result of medication or iodinated radiocontrast agents used in certain types of X-ray procedures.

In healthy people, the amounts of T3 and T4 in the blood are maintained within narrow limits by a hormone known as thyroid-stimulating hormone (TSH) or thyrotropin. TSH is secreted by the anterior pituitary gland, which is a pea-sized structure that extends from the undersurface of the brain just behind the eyes and is enclosed in a bony depression in the base of the skull.

When thyroid disease causes the thyroid hormone levels in the blood to fall, TSH secretion from the pituitary increases; when the thyroid hormone levels rise, TSH secretion switches off in a relationship known as "negative feedback," a concept familiar to engineers and biologists. The feedback of thyroid hormones is magnified ten-fold at the level of the pituitary gland, and, therefore, changes in serum TSH are detectable sooner than changes in thyroid hormone levels.

Maintaining Normal Hormone Levels

The production of thyroid hormones by the thyroid gland is regulated by the pituitary gland, which produces TSH in response to the levels of thyroid hormones in the bloodstream. This mechanism is known as a "negative feedback" loop.

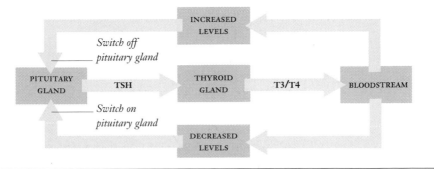

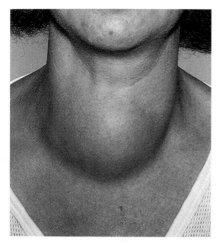

ENLARGED THYROID
Enlargement of the thyroid gland, or goiter, can be caused by iodine deficiency, but this is not a common cause in developed countries.

If your doctor suspects that you may have an underactive thyroid gland, or hypothyroidism, the diagnosis can be confirmed by sending a sample of your blood to a laboratory. If tests show low levels of the hormones T3 and T4 and high levels of TSH in your blood, then your doctor is correct. Similarly, the diagnosis of an overactive thyroid gland or hyperthyroidism would be confirmed by high levels of T3 and T4 and low levels of TSH. The results of the tests are available within a few days.

Patients who suffer from uncomplicated hypothyroidism will not usually be referred to a specialist. Your doctor can prescribe and monitor your treatment. Most patients with hyperthyroidism or with abnormal growth of the thyroid gland will be referred to a specialist for further investigation and advice about treatment.

Thyroid disorders are very common, and hyperthyroidism, hypothyroidism, or abnormal growth or enlargement of the gland, due to diffuse enlargement of one or more thyroid nodules, affects about one in 20 people. Most diseases of the thyroid gland can be treated successfully. Even thyroid cancer may not lead to a reduction in life expectancy if detected early and treated appropriately.

Thyroid disease often runs in families but in an unpredictable manner. Certain forms are associated with an increased risk of developing conditions such as diabetes mellitus or pernicious anemia. All types of thyroid disease are 4–6 times more common in women.

The following chapters will deal with each of the most common thyroid disorders individually.

Incidence of Iodine-deficiency Goiter

This world map shows the regions in which iodine-deficiency goiter is a common disorder. The distribution shows primarily those areas where the soil lacks iodine, and the diet of the people relies entirely on locally produced food.

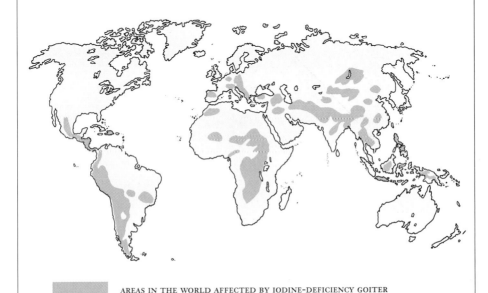

AREAS IN THE WORLD AFFECTED BY IODINE-DEFICIENCY GOITER

Case History: **IODINE DEFICIENCY**

Ahmed was born in a village in the high mountains of northern Pakistan, where he spent most of his childhood. At the age of 20, he came to New York to study engineering. At a routine medical examination, he was found to have a goiter. He felt well, and all the thyroid tests were normal. When Ahmed told the doctor that most of the people in the village where he was born also had a goiter, the cause of the goiter was attributed to iodine deficiency during childhood. His current diet contains enough iodine to prevent the development of hypothyroidism. However, his goiter is likely to remain, even though he has decided to live the rest of his life in a part of the world where there is an adequate amount of iodine in the diet.

KEY POINTS

- Thyroid disease is common, affecting about one in 20 people.
- More women than men are affected.
- Your doctor can diagnose the condition with simple blood tests.
- Treatment is usually successful, and even most types of thyroid cancer can be cured if caught early.

Overactive thyroid

An overactive thyroid, also known as hyperthyroidism or thyrotoxicosis, results from the overproduction of the thyroid hormones T4 and T3 by the thyroid gland. In three-quarters of all patients, this is caused by the presence in the blood of an antibody that stimulates the thyroid to secrete excessive amounts of thyroid hormones and, in some cases, to increase the size of the thyroid gland, producing a goiter.

HYPERTHYROIDISM
Anxiety, palpitations, and a feeling of fullness in the neck are often early symptoms of an overactive thyroid.

This type of hyperthyroidism is known as Graves' disease, named after one of the physicians who described the condition in considerable detail more than 200 years ago.

The cause of the antibody production is not known, but, since Graves' disease runs in families, genes most likely play a part. An environmental factor may trigger the disease in genetically susceptible individuals, but the culprit has not been identified. Stress, in the form of major life events such as divorce or death of a relative, may also precipitate the disease.

Some patients with Graves' disease develop prominent eyes called proptosis or exophthalmos, and a few also suffer from raised, red, itchy areas of skin, known as pretibial myxedema, on the front of the lower legs or top of the feet. These symptoms, like the production of the thyroid-stimulating antibodies, are caused by an abnormality in the patient's immune system that doctors do not yet fully understand.

Most other patients with hyperthyroidism have a goiter containing one or more nodules or "lumps." These nodules also overproduce thyroid hormones; however, unlike the normal thyroid tissue, they are not under the control of thyroid-stimulating hormone, TSH.

Graves' disease can develop at any age but most commonly affects women aged 20–45. Between one-third and one-half of all patients will have a single episode of hyperthyroidism lasting several months. The rest will have successive episodes of hyperthyroidism that will occur over many years. Unfortunately, it is not possible to predict the pattern of hyperthyroidism when it first occurs. Hyperthyroidism resulting from a nodular goiter is unusual before the age of 40. Unlike some patients with Graves' disease, patients with this condition have it indefinitely once it has developed.

Symptoms of an Overactive Thyroid

- Weight loss
- Heat intolerance
- Irritability
- Palpitations
- Breathlessness
- Tremor
- Muscle weakness
- Increase in bowel movements
- Irregular menstruation
- Itchy skin, thinning of the hair, brittle nails
- Watering eyes
- Goiter

HOW DOES IT DEVELOP?

Most patients will have had symptoms for at least six months before they go to see their doctor, but may not realize it. However, in some, usually teenagers, the onset is more rapid, and symptoms are usually noticeable in the first few weeks. Not all patients with hyperthyroidism have all the symptoms listed in the box above. In elderly people, the predominant features, in addition to weight loss, are often a reduction in appetite, muscle weakness, heart failure, apathy, and depression. A young woman, on the other hand, may appear to be full of energy and be unable to sit still for more than a few seconds.

WHAT ARE THE SYMPTOMS?

An overactive thyroid gland causes the chemical reactions in the body to accelerate, producing mental as well as physical symptoms.

WEIGHT LOSS

This happens to almost all patients as a result of a "burning off" of calories caused by the high levels of thyroid hormones in the blood. You will probably find you are hungry all the time and even have to get up during the night to eat. The weight loss can range from 4–7 pounds up to as much as 80 pounds or more. However, a few people find that their appetite increases to such an extent that they may gain a little weight. If you are severely over-weight when the condition first starts, you will probably be delighted to find that you are losing weight and will credit your diet. Unfortunately, you will regain the weight once you are being treated.

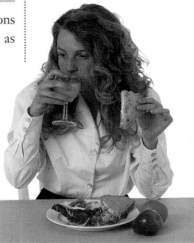

INCREASED APPETITE
People with an overactive thyroid may find that despite eating much more than usual, they still lose weight.

HEAT INTOLERANCE AND SWEATING

As your metabolic rate increases, your body produces excessive heat, which is released by sweating. You will not enjoy warm weather or a centrally heated environment and may be comfortable scantily dressed on a cold winter's day. In extreme cases, your inability to tolerate heat may lead to disagreements with other people as you constantly lower thermostats, open windows, and toss blankets off the bed.

IRRITABILITY

Irritability most often affects women with young families. You may find yourself increasingly unable to cope with the demands and stresses of children, and you may lose your temper frequently and be sensitive to criticism, bursting into tears for no apparent reason.

You may also find it difficult to concentrate, which can adversely affect your performance either in the classroom or at work.

PALPITATIONS

Most patients experience palpitations or are aware of the heart beating at a rate that is faster than normal. In severe, long-standing, untreated hyperthyroidism, particularly in more elderly people, there may be an irregular heartbeat, known as atrial fibrillation, and even heart failure may occur.

SHORTNESS OF BREATH

This is most likely to be noticeable when you exert yourself; for example, after you have climbed two or three short flights of stairs. Individuals who already suffer from asthma may notice a worsening of their symptoms.

SHORTNESS OF BREATH
An overactive thyroid can make you feel breathless, which may be particularly apparent after physical exertion.

TREMOR

Most patients with hyperthyroidism complain of shaky hands. This symptom may be mistaken by friends and relatives for the tremor of alcoholism. You will find it increasingly difficult to hold a cup still or to insert a key into a lock. Your handwriting may deteriorate due to the shakiness of your hands.

MUSCLE WEAKNESS

Characteristically, the thigh muscles become weak, making it hard to climb stairs or to get up from a squatting position or a low chair without using your arms.

BOWEL MOVEMENT CHANGES

There tends to be an increase in the frequency of bowel movements, and a softer-than-normal stool may be passed two or three times daily. Diarrhea can occasionally be a problem.

IRREGULAR MENSTRUAL PERIODS

Menstrual periods are often irregular, light, or even absent. Until the hyperthyroidism has been adequately treated, it may be difficult to conceive.

SKIN, HAIR, AND NAIL PROBLEMS

You may find that your whole body itches. People with Graves' disease, as mentioned earlier, may develop raised itchy patches called pretibial myxedema on their lower legs and feet. Your hair will probably become thinner and finer than usual and will be difficult to style. Your nails will be brittle and become less attractive.

EYE PROBLEMS

People with Graves' disease often have problems with their eyes. These include excessive watering made worse by wind and bright light. Pain and grittiness develop as if there is sand in the eyes. Double vision and blurring of vision also occur. Many sufferers are naturally upset because they develop exophthalmos or protruding eyes as well as "bags" under their eyes.

GOITER

Although often obvious, a goiter is unlikely to cause any symptoms other than a sensation of something unusual in your neck.

HOW IS IT DIAGNOSED?

You will probably have had a blood test taken at your doctor's office, but you may have further blood tests done by an endocrinologist, a specialist in glandular diseases. The specialist or your doctor may also wish to do a thyroid scan to obtain more information about the cause of the hyperthyroidism and how to treat it.

A thyroid scan requires a tiny dose of radioactive iodine or technetium. This will be given either orally or by injection into a vein. The dose is so small that it can even be given to someone who is known to be allergic to iodine. Most specialists, however, try to avoid radioactive scanning in a pregnant or breast-feeding woman.

Sometimes, before a definite diagnosis is made, symptoms may be eased by one of the beta blocker drugs such as propranolol, which counteract to some extent the actions of thyroid hormones. However, beta blockers should not be used by people with asthma.

WHAT IS THE TREATMENT?

There are three forms of treatment for the hyperthyroidism caused by Graves' disease. These are drugs, surgery, and radioactive iodine.

DRUGS

Antithyroid drugs are often given to younger patients who go to their doctor when they have their first episode of hyperthyroidism. One commonly used drug is methimazole, which reduces the amount of hormones made by the thyroid gland. It is available as 5-milligram and 10-milligram tablets. A higher dose (20–30 milligrams daily) is used initially, and your symptoms should start to improve after 14–21 days. Treatment is normally continued for 6–18 months, after which up to half the patients will have recovered and remain well. At the beginning of treatment, your doctor will review your condition every four to six weeks, and the dose of methimazole will be reduced in stages down to 5–15 milligrams daily in a single dose, depending upon the results of measurements of your blood levels of T3, T4, and TSH.

Some specialists prefer to give a high dose of methimazole throughout treatment, usually 30 milligrams daily. If this high dose were to continue for several weeks or more, you would eventually develop an underactive thyroid gland, and therefore levothyroxine is added to the methimazole once thyroid hormone levels have returned to normal. The advantage of this type of treatment is that it does not need to be reviewed as often. It may be beneficial for some patients with severe eye disease, but is no more effective in controlling the symptoms of hyper-thyroidism than methimazole alone.

- **What you should know about drugs** Few people will experience side effects from methimazole. Those rare incidences usually develop within three to four weeks of starting treatment. A skin rash affects five to eight percent of all patients, but the more serious reaction is a reduction in the number of white blood cells, which causes mouth ulcers and infection with a high fever. Your doctor should warn you about these possible effects when you first start the treatment. If you develop adverse effects, you should stop taking the drug and contact your doctor immediately. You may then be prescribed an alternative drug, called propylthiouracil, which works in a similar way to methimazole.

SURGERY

Unfortunately, despite treatment with methimazole or propylthiouracil alone or in combination with levothyroxine for up to 18 months, about half of all patients will develop hyperthyroidism again and usually within two years of stopping the drug. If you are under 45 when you have your second bout of hyperthyroidism, one option is to treat the condition surgically by removing about three-quarters of your thyroid gland.

However, before surgery can be performed, thyroid hormone levels in your blood must be restored to normal with methimazole. Before surgery, you may be asked to take an iodine-containing medication for 10–14 days to reduce the size of the thyroid and its blood flow, which makes the operation technically simpler for the surgeon. You usually go into the hospital the day before your surgery, which lasts about one hour, and return home between two and four days afterward.

• **What you should know about surgery** The main disadvantage is a scar, which usually becomes pale and unnoticeable among the skin creases in the neck. You can also wear jewelry or scarves to hide it. In very rare cases (less than one percent), the parathyroid glands, which lie close to the thyroid and control the level of calcium in the blood, may be damaged, in which case long-term treatment with oral vitamin D will be necessary. Equally rare is damage to one of the nerves supplying the voice box, which may result in significant alteration to the quality of the voice. Although not critical to some people, the voice change could make surgery a less acceptable option to those who depend upon their voice for a living.

The initial results of surgery performed by an experienced doctor are good. Eighty percent of sufferers will be cured immediately. However, 15 percent will have had too much thyroid tissue removed and will become hypothyroid; 5 percent will have had insufficient thyroid tissue removed and remain hyperthyroid. These failures are not the result of surgical incompetence but have more to do with the nature of the underlying thyroid disease. Furthermore, in time, an increasing proportion of those patients whose hyperthyroidism was originally cured by surgery will develop an underactive thyroid gland. Recurrence of hyperthyroidism may even develop 20–40 years after apparently successful surgery. If the condition recurs, performing a second operation is unusual because repeat surgery is technically difficult and the risk of damage to the surrounding structures in the neck increases.

LITTLE TO SHOW
The scar left by thyroid surgery soon fades and becomes indistinct. There is then no need to cover the neck with scarves or jewelry.

RADIOACTIVE IODINE (IODINE-131)

Radioactive iodine is currently the treatment of choice in the US. Traditionally, this form of treatment was reserved for patients over age 40–45 and beyond child-bearing age or for younger individuals who had been sterilized. This conservative approach was originally adopted because of concern that radioactive iodine might lead to birth defects in children conceived after the treatment. In fact, there is no evidence for birth defects. Consequently, in some hospitals there has been a move toward using radioactive iodine in a wider range of patients because it is inexpensive, easy to administer, and effective.

Radioactive iodine is taken as a capsule or a drink that tastes like water and is usually administered in a radiology department. Before receiving treatment, you may be asked to sign a consent form and should receive instructions about avoiding close contact with people, including young children, for a few days after therapy. Radioactive iodine is never prescribed for pregnant women because it will adversely affect the fetal thyroid gland. Women are advised not to conceive until three to four months after treatment.

Radioactive iodine destroys some of the thyroid cells and prevents other cells from dividing, which is how they are normally replaced at the end of their lifespan. The treatment takes 6–16 weeks to work. In the interim, depending upon the severity of the hyperthyroidism, you may be given propranolol or methimazole to relieve your symptoms. Six to eight weeks following treatment, you will need a checkup. If you are one of the minority of people who is still hyperthyroid after four to six months, you will be given a second dose of radioactive iodine.

• **What you should know about radioactive iodine** The major problem with this treatment is the development of hypothyroidism, which is most likely to appear in the first year after treatment, affecting at least 50 percent of people. In each subsequent year, two to four percent of people will be affected. The great majority become hypothyroid eventually. Therefore, you should have regular checkups either with a specialist or with your primary care doctor.

The treatment for hypothyroidism is levothyroxine in a dose of 100–150 micrograms daily. Levothyroxine does not cause side effects if the appropriate dose is taken regularly.

Considering Which Treatment Is Right for You

An overactive thyroid may be treated with drugs, radioactive iodine, or surgery. Choice of treatment depends on the individual patient. All options should be discussed with a specialist.

- No treatment is perfect. Discuss the options with your specialist. Some patients do not want surgery, even when a course of antithyroid drugs has failed.
- A second, or even a third, course of drugs can be used in the hope that the disease will ultimately "burn itself out." Indeed, before treatment existed for the hyperthyroidism of Graves' disease, some patients got better spontaneously after months or years and then became hypothyroid.
- Some patients dislike the idea of radioactive iodine treatment. Some specialists believe surgery is the best treatment for a young patient with severe hyperthyroidism and a large goiter.
- Whatever kind of treatment you have for hyperthyroidism, you will need regular follow-up appointments, including an annual blood test.

Case History 1: **HEART SYMPTOMS**

Although 70-year-old John Parry considered himself to be generally very healthy, he recently noticed his ankles swelling. At first, the swelling was just at night, but then it became noticeable all the time. His legs felt very heavy. One night he woke up at 1 a.m., gasping for breath and coughing up frothy white sputum. His wife called an ambulance. Mr. Parry was admitted to the local hospital within 20 minutes. The doctor on duty, Dr. Mackenzie, correctly diagnosed heart failure as the cause of the fluid accumulation in John's legs and lungs. He also noticed that John's pulse was very rapid and irregular. An electrocardiogram indicated the abnormal pulse was caused by atrial fibrillation. John was given oxygen with a face mask, an injection of a drug called furosemide to get rid of the excess fluid, and digoxin pills to reduce the speed of his heartbeat. Since patients with atrial fibrillation have an increased risk of forming blood clots in the heart, which can break loose and result in a stroke or a blocked artery in a leg, the drug warfarin was given to thin the blood.

Dr. Mackenzie knew that atrial fibrillation could sometimes occur as a complication of an overactive thyroid gland, particularly in older patients.

Mr. Parry did have hyperthyroidism, which turned out to be caused by Graves' disease. He was treated with radioactive iodine. He was also given the antithyroid drug, methimazole, for six weeks until the radioactive iodine had time to take effect.

At first, Mr. Parry was concerned about the number of pills he was taking after his hospital stay. However, the medications were all stopped within six months as his thyroid gland came under control. Mr. Parry's heart is now beating regularly, and he is as fit as ever. His doctor orders blood tests regularly to test the thyroid hormone levels and make sure that Mr. Parry is not developing an underactive thyroid gland as a result of the radioactive iodine treatment.

Case History 2: **RECURRENT SYMPTOMS**

Anna Robinson had had a previous episode of hyper-thyroidism caused by Graves' disease in her mid-twenties, for which she had been given an 18-month course of methimazole. At the age of 45, she was troubled by the heat but attributed the symptom to menopause.

However, she began to lose weight, and her hands became shaky. She realized that her thyroid gland was overactive again. An endocrinologist suggested radioactive iodine treatment. In spite of reassurances and the evidence that this form of treatment was not associated with any risk other than the eventual onset of an underactive thyroid gland, Mrs. Robinson was uneasy.

She was aware of various articles in the media suggesting a possible link between radiation and leukemia in people living near nuclear power plants. She did not like the idea of having to avoid her new granddaughter, even if for only a few days after treatment.

Also, since she sang in the local church choir, thyroid surgery was inappropriate because of the possibility of a change in the quality of her voice.

Mrs. Robinson was relieved to learn that she could be treated with methimazole again.

GRAVES' DISEASE AND THE EYES

The signs of Graves' disease that affect the eyes are known as ophthalmopathy or orbitopathy and are present in most patients if a doctor looks closely enough. Sometimes the signs occur before the onset of the overactive thyroid gland or after the successful treatment of the hyperthyroidism. One eye is often affected more than the other.

An early sign is retraction of the upper eyelid, which appears as if it has been pulled up, exposing more of the white of the eye and causing a staring appearance. This may improve after the elevated levels of thyroid hormone have been restored to normal with treatment. Some patients complain of dry, gritty eyes, as if there were sand in them, and of constant blinking or excessive watering.

The other features of thyroid eye disease result from a buildup of pressure behind the eyeball, which sits in a bony socket called the orbit. The space between the eyeball and the back of the orbit contains the muscles that move the eye; the optic nerve, which relays messages to the brain; and fat.

In patients with thyroid eye disease, excessive amounts of water accumulate behind the eyeball, and the muscles and fat become swollen and spongy. The muscles increase in bulk two- or threefold and cease to work efficiently.

As a result, the normal movement of the eyes may be restricted and uncomfortable, with double vision, or diplopia, and even development of crossed eyes. The increase in pressure behind the eyeballs pushes them forward, producing the "bug-eyed" appearance known as exophthalmos or proptosis. The increased exposure of the eyeballs makes them more prone to irritation from dust, grit, wind, and sun. The cornea may also be damaged. In addition, some of the fat behind the eyeballs may be forced into the eyelids, contributing to their puffiness and the appearance of "bags under the eyes." Very rarely, in severely affected patients, the increased pressure may damage the optic nerve and cause partial or total loss of vision.

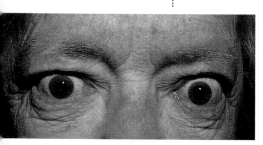

PROTRUDING EYES
Most patients with Graves' disease suffer some form of eye disorder. Bulging eyeballs, causing a staring appearance, are a common sign.

Treatment of the eye disease is not as satisfactory as that of the overactive thyroid gland. Smoking is thought to make the eye disease worse, as does poor control of hyperthyroidism. It is very important, therefore, that you stop smoking entirely and follow carefully your doctor's instructions about dosage of medications such as methimazole or levothyroxine. If you have dry eyes or even excessive watering, a prescription for artificial tears may relieve the symptoms. Wearing dark glasses in sunny weather may also help.

Less Common Types of Hyperthyroidism

Occasionally, an overactive thyroid may be caused by a viral infection or by treatment with a particular drug.

- Mild hyperthyroidism, lasting for a few weeks, may occur after a viral infection of the thyroid; this is known as viral or de Quervain's thyroiditis. The most prominent feature is severe pain and tenderness over the thyroid gland associated with symptoms of a flulike illness. The hyperthyroidism rarely needs any treatment other than a beta blocking drug, such as propranolol. An equally short-lived period of mild hypothyroidism usually follows and then full recovery.

- The iodine-containing drug, amiodarone, which is used increasingly by heart specialists for the treatment of certain irregularities of heart rhythm, may cause hyperthyroidism. Your blood thyroid levels should be checked before you start taking the drug and at six-month intervals while you are on it.

- Nodular goiter: This condition is treated either with surgery or with radioactive iodine. Unlike someone with Graves' disease, you are less likely to develop hypothyroidism. At one time, thyroxine was routinely prescribed after surgery to prevent regrowth of the goiter, which is common over a subsequent period of about 20 years. However, this drug is not really useful unless you develop hypothyroidism, and it has not been shown to effectively diminish the site of the thyroid.

Patients who are experiencing more advanced thyroid disease that threatens vision may require treatment with a steroid drug, such as prednisolone, which reduces the poorly understood processes that lead to accumulation of water behind the eyeball. In some cases, radiation therapy has been used with some success in the treatment of thyroid eye disease. An operation may be required to remove part of the wall of the orbit, thereby reducing the pressure behind the eyeball.

Major surgery is rarely necessary, however, and would be performed only after close collaboration between your thyroid and eye specialists. Most people who have Graves' disease discover that their eye problems settle down considerably over a period of two to three years. At that stage, relatively minor surgery will correct double vision as well as reduce the "staring" look and the bags under the eyes.

Some evidence suggests that the eye disease may deteriorate after treatment with radioactive iodine for hyperthyroidism. Some specialists will not prescribe this form of therapy for anyone whose eyes are badly affected.

EYE PROBLEMS
Artificial tears may help if you suffer from dry or excessively watery eyes, a common complaint with thyroid disorders.

KEY POINTS

- About three-quarters of all cases of hyperthyroidism are caused by Graves' disease.
- Graves' disease may be inherited. However, other factors are also involved in triggering the condition.
- The people most likely to develop Graves' disease are women between the ages of 20 and 45.
- Graves' disease can be treated by drugs, surgery, and radioactive iodine. No one treatment is right for everyone.
- Discuss treatment options with your specialist before making the final decision on which approach is best.
- After treatment, regular checkups are necessary to make sure that you stay well.
- Most people with Graves' disease experience some eye problems, which may be only minor irritations. More serious symptoms can be treated and usually disappear over time.

Underactive thyroid

CHECKING THE THYROID
Your doctor will feel your thyroid gland to determine its size and consistency.

An underactive thyroid, or hypothyroidism, occurs when the thyroid gland stops producing enough of the thyroid hormones T3 and T4. In its most common form, affecting one percent of the population, the thyroid gland shrinks as its cells are all destroyed by a subtle defect in the patient's immune system. Middle-aged and elderly women are the most commonly affected.

Hypothyroidism may be caused by simple underactivity of the thyroid gland or a defect in the immune system. If it is due to a defect in the immune system, which also leads to an enlargement of the thyroid and the formation of a goiter, it is known as Hashimoto's thyroiditis. Both of these types of hypothyroidism are associated, as is Graves' disease, with the other autoimmune diseases (see box, p.32). Although having hypothyroidism makes you more likely to develop more autoimmune conditions than other people, the risk is still small. Hypothyroidism may also result from treatment for Graves' disease with either surgery or radioactive iodine.

HOW DOES IT DEVELOP?

Hypothyroidism does not come on overnight, but slowly over many months. You may not notice the symptoms at first or may simply associate them with aging.

Primary care physicians have easy access to laboratory tests for hypothyroidism. As a result, hypothyroidism is increasingly likely to be diagnosed at a relatively early stage when symptoms are mild. Hypothyroidism in its advanced state is sometimes known as myxedema.

It would be unusual to have all the symptoms mentioned below unless the diagnosis had been delayed for some reason for months or even years. You are more likely to go to your doctor with rather vague complaints such as fatigue and weight gain, which could be due to a variety of causes.

If a blood test shows that you have low T4 and high thyroid-stimulating hormone (TSH) levels, hypothyroidism is confirmed. Unless there is a complication, such as angina, your treatment can be managed by your primary care physician.

WHAT ARE THE SYMPTOMS?

Underactivity of the thyroid gland slows down the chemical reactions in the body, causing the following:

WEIGHT GAIN

Most patients gain 3–10 pounds, even though appetite is normal or even less than usual.

SENSITIVITY TO THE COLD

You may feel the cold more readily than other people, want to wear extra layers of clothing, and sit close to a heater. You may also suffer from muscle stiffness

Associated Diseases

Although the risk is small, an underactive thyroid can lead to an increased likelihood of developing one of the following autoimmune diseases:

- Pernicious anemia: regular injections of vitamin B$_{12}$ are necessary to maintain a normal blood count.
- Diabetes mellitus: a condition that usually requires treatment with insulin.
- Addison's disease: the adrenal glands, which sit on top of each kidney, produce insufficient cortisol and aldosterone, hormones that can be replaced orally.
- Premature ovarian failure: this causes loss of menstrual periods, infertility, and early menopause.
- Underactivity of the parathyroid glands (glands adjacent to the thyroid): this leads to a low level of calcium in the blood and to a nervous condition called tetany, which is effectively treated with vitamin D capsules.
- Vitiligo: this is a skin disease in which there are areas of loss of pigmentation, giving a bleached appearance.

and spasm when you move suddenly, especially when it is cold.

MENTAL PROBLEMS

You may feel tired or sleepy and slow down intellectually, and your reactions may slow. Fortunately, however, your sense of humor is unaffected. Older patients may be incorrectly thought to be suffering from dementia, while some people experience depression and paranoia, which are the basis for what is called "myxedema madness."

SLURRED SPEECH

Your voice becomes slow and husky. Speech is often slurred.

HEART PROBLEMS

In contrast to a person with an overactive thyroid gland, the pulse rate of someone who has hypothyroidism is slow, about 60 beats per minute or less. You may have high blood pressure. An elderly patient with severe long-standing hypothyroidism is at risk of heart failure. Angina can be the first symptom of hypothyroidism.

CONSTIPATION

As the result of the general slowing down of the body's processes, you may suffer from constipation.

HEAVY MENSTRUAL PERIODS

Your menstrual periods become heavier if you have not yet reached menopause.

SKIN AND HAIR PROBLEMS

The skin is likely to become pale, course, and dry, and to flake easily. Eyelids, hands, and feet tend to swell. Some people may find their skin has a lemon-yellowish tint. Prominent blood vessels in the cheeks may cause a purplish flush. Some people experience loss of skin pigmentation known as vitiligo. Your hair may become dry and brittle, and the outer part of your eyebrows may fall out.

NERVOUS SYSTEM DISORDERS

You may become a little deaf and have trouble with your balance. If your fingers tingle, particularly during the night, you may find that shaking your hands vigorously provides relief. Tingling of the fingers may also be caused by pinching of one of the nerves that supplies the hand as it travels through the wrist (carpal tunnel syndrome).

WHAT IS THE TREATMENT?

Hypothyroidism is treated with levothyroxine. Normally, treatment starts slowly. You will be prescribed an initial daily dose of 25–50 micrograms for a few weeks. The dose is then adjusted based on your blood test results. It should not be adjusted more frequently than every six to eight weeks. The aim is to restore levels of T4 and TSH in the blood to normal.

You should start to feel better within two to three weeks and notice the puffiness around your eyes disappearing.

However, your skin and hair texture may take three to six months to recover fully. Normally you will need levothyroxine treatment for life.

Case History: **SUDDEN FALL IN GLUCOSE LEVELS**

Jean Spencer was 17 and in her final year of high school, planning to go to college. She had been diagnosed with type 1 diabetes at age 11 and gave herself insulin injections twice each day. Control of her diabetes had always been satisfactory, and her dose of insulin did not vary much. She had been puzzled for three months, however, because she did not seem to require as much insulin as before. On four occasions she had almost lost consciousness in class because of a low level of glucose in her blood but had been revived with sugary drinks by her teacher.

One time, however, she did not respond, and was rushed to the local hospital, given intravenous glucose, and kept overnight. Jean's parents and her teacher were also concerned because she was not concentrating in class, and her schoolwork had not been as good as usual. She had also begun to complain of the cold, and she had not been able to sing in the school Christmas concert because her voice had become husky. Her aunt, who was visiting from Canada, recognized the change in Jean's appearance since her last visit the previous year.

Jean's aunt had developed

JEAN'S TREATMENT
Seen here testing her blood sugar levels, Jean noticed a change in the effects of her insulin dose. This proved to be caused by an underactive thyroid, which was treated with levothyroxine.

an underactive thyroid gland 10 years earlier and suggested to Jean that she have a blood test. Jean is now taking levothyroxine, like her aunt, and her insulin dose has returned to its previous level. She graduated from high school with honors and is now in her first semester at college.

SPECIAL SITUATIONS

The level of various fats or lipids in the blood is increased in hypothyroidism. In some people with long-standing hypothyroidism and increased lipids, the coronary arteries can become narrowed by fatty deposits. Insufficient blood reaches the heart muscle, especially during exercise, and the sufferer may experience pain in the middle of the chest, known as angina.

Treatment with levothyroxine may also worsen angina. Someone with angina will be started on a lower dose, and increases will be made more slowly than usual. It may be necessary to treat the cause of the abnormal blood flow to the coronary arteries before or after starting treatment. Levothyroxine dosage should also be carefully monitored during pregnancy (see p.41).

TEMPORARY HYPOTHYROIDISM

It is usually necessary for treatment with levothyroxine to be continued throughout the patient's life. However, if you develop hypothyroidism in the first three to four months after surgery or radioactive iodine treatment for Graves' disease it may be short-lived, lasting only a few weeks. You may not need any treatment. The same is true for the hypothyroidism that occurs as a complication of postpartum thyroiditis (see p.43) or de Quervain's thyroiditis (see p.27).

SUBCLINICAL HYPOTHYROIDISM

Most doctors will arrange for someone to have a blood test even when they suspect thyroid problems. However, minor abnormalities can be detected in patients who visit their doctor because of a variety of vague symptoms, such as fatigue, or in people who have a family history of autoimmune disease.

The most common finding is the combination of a "normal" T4 and a raised TSH level, known to doctors as subclinical hypothyroidism. Five to 20 percent of these people will develop more obvious hypothyroidism in each subsequent year. For this reason, depending on the symptoms, some doctors prescribe levothyroxine for subclinical hypothyroidism. This may have a dramatic effect on the individual's symptoms.

DRUG-RELATED HYPOTHYROIDISM

Lithium, which is widely used for bipolar disorder, may cause goiter and hypothyroidism. When, as normally happens, a person needs extended treatment with lithium, treatment with levothyroxine will also be necessary.

Amiodarone, which is used in the treatment of certain heart irregularities, may cause either hyperthyroidism or hypothyroidism. Anyone on this drug will need thyroid blood tests periodically.

KEY POINTS

- Hypothyroidism usually comes on slowly, and symptoms are likely to be vague at first.
- Your doctor will be able to confirm the diagnosis with a simple blood test.
- Lifelong treatment may be necessary.
- Some people who have been hypothyroid for years may suffer from chest pain due to angina. Since levothyroxine can aggravate angina, the dosage will need monitoring. If you already have angina when your thyroid condition is discovered, treatment will be adjusted accordingly.
- If your thyroid blood test is only slightly abnormal, you may be given preventive treatment with levothyroxine.

Thyroid disease and pregnancy

It is important to tell your doctor that you are planning to become pregnant if you suffer from any kind of thyroid disease. Your doctor will want to keep your thyroid hormone levels under careful control throughout the pregnancy to prevent harm to the baby.

GRAVES' DISEASE

Hyperthyroidism occurring during pregnancy is almost always the result of Graves' disease, but it is not common. Autoimmune diseases such as Graves' disease tend to improve on their own during pregnancy. Women with an overactive thyroid gland are relatively infertile because a greater proportion of their menstrual cycles do not release an egg from the ovaries. Failure to recognize hyperthyroidism or to treat it adequately in a pregnant woman may lead to miscarriage.

Since the thyroid-stimulating antibody that is responsible for the hyperthyroidism of Graves' disease crosses the placenta and passes from the blood of the mother to that of the developing child, the fetus may develop an overactive thyroid gland like its mother.

DRUGS AND PREGNANCY
Close control of the activity of the thyroid gland is important during pregnancy.

Fortunately, antithyroid drugs also cross the placenta and good control of hyperthyroidism in the mother will ensure that the fetus remains unharmed. However, over-treatment with antithyroid drugs may lead to development of a goiter in the fetus.

It is important, therefore, that the patient be prescribed the lowest dose of methimazole possible to restore thyroid hormone levels in the blood to normal. The levels of thyroid hormones must be checked every four to six weeks, in close cooperation with the patient's obstetrician. Treatment with methimazole is usually stopped four weeks before the expected date of delivery to make sure that the fetus is not hypothyroid at a crucial time in its development.

If hyperthyroidism recurs in a breast-feeding mother after the baby is born, she should be treated with propylthiouracil rather than methimazole because the small amount excreted in the milk will not affect the baby.

Some reports in the US indicate that methimazole may be associated with a rare disease in the newborn baby, known as aplasia cutis, which is a defect in the skin covering a small part of the scalp. However, this risk may be overestimated, if it is present at all. Many specialists prescribe methimazole during pregnancy. Others may prefer to use propylthiouracil or to change from methi-mazole before conception if possible. The dose of propylthiouracil is ten times that of methimazole and is available as 50 milligram tablets only.

Radioactive iodine treatment is never given during pregnancy. Surgery is occasionally advised around week 20 of pregnancy for patients who develop side effects to the drugs for Graves' disease or who take them irregularly, thereby putting the fetus at risk.

HYPERTHYROIDISM IN THE NEWBORN

In most women with Graves' disease, the thyroid-stimulating antibody disappears during pregnancy, or its level in the blood becomes low. In some, however, the antibody level remains high. Since the maternal antibody can cross the placenta throughout pregnancy, these high levels are also present in the blood of the newborn and may cause hyperthyroidism. It is possible to predict which babies are most likely to develop hyperthyroidism by finding high levels of antibodies in the mother's blood toward the end of pregnancy. Hyperthyroidism in the newborn, if detected at this stage, is easily treated and lasts only two to three weeks until the antibody from the mother is broken down and inactivated. Rarely, mothers who have been treated successfully for Graves' disease in the past continue to produce thyroid-stimulating antibody, and their newborn offspring are at risk of developing hyperthyroidism.

All newborn babies in the US have a blood test shortly after birth to detect deficiency of thyroid hormone, a separate condition (see p.42).

Case History 1: **CONCEPTION AND PREGNANCY**

Rebecca and her husband had been trying to have a second child for three years without success. Rebecca had conceived twice but unfortunately had miscarried on each occasion at about ten weeks. She felt and looked well. Although she had lost a few pounds in weight, Rebecca attributed this to her busy lifestyle of running a home, looking after an active five-year-old son, and working part-time as a secretary. She was a little anxious that her menstrual periods, which used to be regular, had become much lighter and occasionally were missed.

During a telephone call to her mother, she learned that her cousin in Australia had recently been diagnosed with an overactive thyroid gland. She consulted her doctor. Despite a lack of obvious signs, such as a goiter or bulging eyes, Rebecca had mild hyperthyroidism, confirmed by blood tests, and further tests indicated that it was due to Graves' disease. Treatment was started with methimazole, initially in a dose of 30 milligrams daily. After five months of treatment, Rebecca was pregnant again.

She was seen by an endocrinologist every four weeks, and, by the middle of her pregnancy, she required only 5 milligrams of methimazole every day. The drug was stopped four weeks before the expected date of delivery. Rebecca gave birth to a healthy girl whose heel-prick blood test at seven days showed no evidence of thyroid abnormality. Rebecca breast-fed her daughter but, after six months, developed hyperthyroidism due to recurrent Graves' disease. She decided to change to bottle-feeding. Her hyperthyroidism was then treated with methimazole as before. Had she opted to continue breast-feeding, propylthiouracil would have been prescribed instead.

TAKING A SAMPLE
In Rebecca's case, blood tests showed that she was suffering from mild hyperthyroidism, which was increasing her chances of having a miscarriage.

HYPOTHYROIDISM

Most patients with hypothyroidism are already taking levothyroxine when they become pregnant. Although mild hypothyroidism is unlikely to reduce fertility, patients with severe thyroid deficiency of long duration are unlikely to become pregnant or, if they conceive, to maintain their pregnancy.

The dose of levothyroxine may need to be increased during pregnancy by as much as 50–75 micrograms daily. Blood tests should be performed every three months to check whether the dose needs to be increased. The dose taken before pregnancy can be resumed three to four weeks after childbirth. The thyroid gland of the fetus develops independently of the mother and makes its own hormones. Therefore, the baby will not be at risk if you forget the occasional dose of levothyroxine, but making a habit of not taking it increases the chances of miscarriage.

HYPOTHYROIDISM IN THE NEWBORN

One in about 3,500 newborn babies has an underactive thyroid gland as a result of failure of the gland to develop normally. In the past, the problem was not recognized until the child was several weeks or months old, by which time he or she would have been likely to develop permanent mental and physical handicap, a condition known then as cretinism. Today, however, all newborn babies are screened by a blood test for hypothyroidism between five and seven days after birth. Affected children are given prompt treatment that ensures normal development. Treatment usually continues throughout life. In a few babies, however, the hypothyroidism is temporary. Temporary hypothyroidism is a result of being born to a mother with an underactive thyroid gland, in whom blocking antibodies cross the placenta and have the opposite effect of the stimulating antibodies that produce Graves' disease and neonatal hyperthyroidism (see p.40).

HYPOTHYROIDISM IN BABIES
A simple pinprick test on the heel is performed on all newborn babies to test for hypothyroidism.

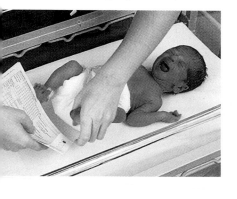

AFTER CHILDBIRTH

Although the hyperthyroidism of Graves' disease tends to improve on its own during pregnancy, it often returns in a severe form within a few months of delivery. There is, however, another form of hyperthyroidism that may develop in the first year after childbirth, almost always in mothers who have an underlying autoimmune thyroid disease such as Hashimoto's thyroiditis, which may not have been recognized previously. The hyperthyroidism is mild, lasts only a few weeks, and can be treated with a beta blocker if necessary. This phase may be followed by an equally transient episode of mild hypothyroidism not requiring treatment, which is then usually followed by full recovery. A similar pattern may occur in future pregnancies, and many patients ultimately develop a permanently underactive thyroid.

It is important to distinguish between this condition, known as postpartum thyroiditis, which does not require treatment, and Graves' disease, which does. To do so, it may be necessary to evaluate the ability of the thyroid gland to concentrate radioactive iodine or technetium, which is lacking in postpartum thyroiditis. Postpartum thyroiditis affects about five percent of women, but most patients do not experience symptoms. There does not appear to be any association between these thyroid blood test abnormalities and postpartum depression.

Case History 2: POSTPARTUM THYROIDITIS

Flora Stewart was 25 and happily married to her lawyer husband, William, when they had their first child, Jane. Five months later, their relationship began to deteriorate when Flora became weepy and short-tempered, snapping at William for no reason.

Flora was also sleeping poorly, and William noticed that Flora's hands sometimes trembled. However, they both attributed this to hormonal changes following the birth of their baby and assumed that before long everything would return to normal.

However, when Flora began to complain of palpitations, William persuaded her to see their doctor. The doctor thought that Flora might have an overactive thyroid gland, and his suspicions were confirmed by a blood test.

On hearing the news, Flora was concerned because her mother had suffered from Graves' disease when she was in her thirties. Her mother's eyes were still very prominent 20 years later, even though the hyperthyroidism had been cured. In order to relieve some of Flora's symptoms, her doctor prescribed a long-acting form of propranolol in a dose of 80 milligrams to be taken once daily. He also suggested that Flora see an endocrinologist. By the time of her appointment four weeks later, Flora felt much better, and a blood sample showed that her thyroid gland had become only slightly underactive. The diagnosis was not Graves' disease but postpartum thyroiditis. Flora was reassured that she would not get bulging eyes like her mother. The propranolol was stopped, and another blood test two months later was entirely normal.

Flora now knows that she may get the symptoms of postpartum thyroiditis after further pregnancies and that she has an increased chance of developing a permanently underactive thyroid gland at some stage in the future.

However, her doctor will do a thyroid blood test every year to make sure that the condition is detected before she can develop severe symptoms.

KEY POINTS

- If you are planning a baby and have thyroid disease, tell your doctor because you may need to change drugs.
- If you have thyroid disease, your doctor will keep a close watch on you during pregnancy to assure that your treatment will not harm your developing baby.
- After having a baby, some women will develop mild thyroid disease, which is usually easily treated.
- All newborns are routinely tested for hypothyroidism so that treatment can be started early if needed.

Enlarged thyroid

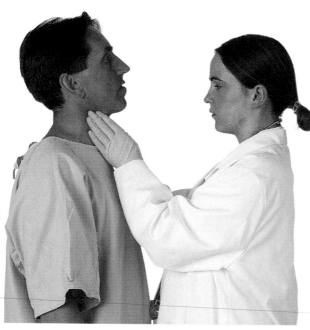

An enlarged thyroid gland is known as a goiter. There are many causes, including a shortage of iodine in the diet, which occurs in remote mountainous parts of the world; drugs such as lithium carbonate used to treat patients with bipolar disorder; and autoimmune disorders such as Hashimoto's thyroiditis (see p.30) and Graves' disease (see pp.13-29).

ASSESSING THE THYROID
Your doctor will usually be able to confirm the presence of a goiter by examining your neck.

The cause of most goiters in the US is not known. Such goiters are called "simple goiters," despite the fact that there are almost certainly complex reasons for their development. Despite being enlarged, the thyroid gland continues to produce normal amounts of hormones, and the patient is referred to as "euthyroid" as opposed to hyperthyroid or hypothyroid. At first, in teenagers and young adults, the goiter is evenly or diffusely enlarged. In some cases, during the next 15 to 25 years, the thyroid continues to grow but becomes full of lumps or nodules.

By the time the person reaches middle age, the goiter is lumpy and is known medically as a "multinodular goiter."

SIMPLE DIFFUSE GOITER

Most of those who have a simple diffuse goiter are young women between the ages of 15 and 25. If you have the condition, you may notice a symmetrical, smooth swelling in the front of your neck. You may have had it for some years but thought it was just "baby fat." The goiter will move up and down when you swallow. It is not tender, however, and does not usually cause difficulty in swallowing. However, you may experience a tight sensation in your neck. The goiter may vary slightly in size and be more noticeable during a menstrual period or pregnancy. It is not normally a cosmetic problem unless it becomes very large.

HOW IS IT DIAGNOSED?

The diagnosis is usually clear from a careful examination of your neck by your doctor, who may refer you to a specialist for additional tests to exclude rarer causes of goiter.

WHAT IS THE TREATMENT?

No treatment is necessary for simple diffuse goiter. In the past, iodine or levothyroxine pills were given, but neither is predictably effective in reducing the size of the gland. Many people find that the goiter becomes less noticeable or even disappears over a period of two to three years.

SIMPLE MULTINODULAR GOITER

If you are middle-aged and have simple multinodular goiter, you will probably become aware of a swelling in your neck while washing or applying makeup in front of a mirror. In fact, the goiter will have been present for many years but either has now reached a critical size or is now obvious because your neck has become thinner. The goiter is often more obvious on one side of the neck than the other. It may vary in size, from being barely visible to being so large that you feel you have to hide it with clothing. A few people first notice the enlarged thyroid gland when internal bleeding causes increased swelling, which is accompanied by bruiselike discomfort in the neck lasting a few days.

If the goiter is large, it may be difficult to swallow dry, solid food. If the goiter impinges on the trachea or windpipe, breathing may be difficult. Singers, in particular, notice a change in their voice.

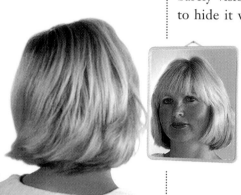

BECOMING AWARE
Many people first notice that they have developed a goiter when looking in the mirror.

HOW IS IT DIAGNOSED?

Your doctor will examine you and may take a blood sample to check that your thyroid hormone levels are normal and may ask a specialist for advice about further investigations and treatment.

Your primary doctor or the specialist may wish to carry out one or more of the following tests:

● **X-rays and breathing tests** These investigations will reveal whether the goiter is compressing or squashing the trachea.

● **Ultrasound scan** A probe, the size of a small flashlight, is passed over the skin of the front of the neck and an image of the goiter is formed on a screen. In addition to showing the goiter's size and extent, the scan also highlights any cysts or nodules that the specialist may not have seen when examining the neck.

• **Isotope scan** This technique provides a different type of image that indicates whether the nodules in the goiter are likely to produce thyroid hormones, in which case the development of an overactive thyroid is more likely in future years. It is obtained by giving a tiny amount of a radioactive substance, technetium-99m or iodine-123. Later, you lie under a sophisticated form of camera for a few minutes to produce an image.

• **Fine needle aspiration** This involves attaching a needle, about the same size as one used for taking a blood sample, to the end of a syringe. Then, while you are lying down, the needle is passed, with or without local anesthesia, through the skin of the neck into the enlarged thyroid gland. Sometimes, this process is done under ultrasound guidance. The discomfort is no greater than a blood test. By pulling on the plunger and moving the needle up and down a tiny distance within the goiter, the doctor can obtain thyroid cells for analysis. These are smeared onto a glass slide and, after processing in the pathology laboratory, are examined under a microscope. The appearance of the cells will help determine whether the thyroid enlargement is the result of a malignant tumor.

Fine needle aspiration, also known as FNA, is not often carried out in patients with a multinodular goiter unless the gland is much bigger on one side than the other, or a portion of the goiter is growing very rapidly. This technique is more often used to evaluate a single or especially promi-nent nodule.

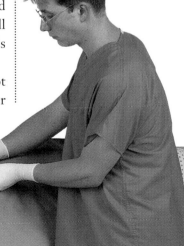

FINE NEEDLE ASPIRATION
In this test, a needle is inserted into the thyroid gland to extract a sample of thyroid cells for analysis.

WHAT IS THE TREATMENT?

If your goiter is relatively small, you probably will not need any treatment. Your doctor will check thyroid hormone levels in your blood every one to two years to be sure that you are not developing hyperthyroidism. Although levothyroxine pills are prescribed in certain parts of the world in an attempt to shrink the goiter, they are not always effective.

If the goiter becomes so large that it is unattractive or if it is compressing the windpipe, the most effective treatment is an operation that removes most of the thyroid gland.

No treatment is necessary before surgery, and you will be in the hospital for about three days. The complications are the same as those for surgery for Graves' disease (see pp.20–21). You may need levothyroxine treatment afterward because there may be insufficient thyroid tissue left to produce adequate amounts of hormones.

In patients who are not healthy enough for surgery or who do not want to have an operation, it may be possible to reduce the size of the goiter by about 50 percent by treating it with radioactive iodine. A large dose is necessary, which may require a 24–48-hour stay in the hospital. If so, you will be given a single room in order to avoid contaminating other patients or visitors with radioactivity. It may take several months for the goiter to shrink. It is unlikely that the thyroid gland will become underactive. The radioactive iodine is primarily concentrated within the nodules, which become smaller. The previously dormant thyroid tissue surrounding the nodules is unaffected by the radiation and may become active and start to produce thyroid hormones.

Case History: **OVERACTIVE THYROID GLAND**

Jenny Morris was a single woman in her seventies who had been an accomplished actress. She always wore a silk scarf around her neck, day and night, summer and winter. Friends and neighbors thought the scarf was part of her slightly eccentric personality. However, when she was rushed to the hospital with abdominal pain due to gallstones, the scarf was removed to reveal a large goiter and a scar from previous thyroid surgery.

Ms. Morris explained that the operation had been carried out for a goiter when she was quite young. In her mid-forties the goiter had appeared again. She had been told that further surgery was out of the question because a second operation would be technically more difficult and any damage to the nearby nerve supply to the voice box or larynx would ruin her stage career. As time passed, the goiter had gradually grown, and she had worn the scarves to avoid embarrassment.

Blood tests in the hospital indicated a slightly over-active thyroid gland. Three months after treatment with radioactive iodine, Jenny's blood level returned to normal. Equally important, a year later, the size of the goiter had been reduced by at least one-half, and she happily abandoned her scarves!

SINGLE THYROID NODULES

Single lumps or nodules in the thyroid are common and can occur at any age. Women are more likely to be affected than men.

A single thyroid nodule varies in size from that of a pea to a golf ball or even larger. Like a goiter, the nodule is usually discovered by accident while washing or looking in a mirror. Bleeding into the nodule may cause pain that may alert you to its presence. Alternatively, the nodule may be discovered during a medical examination for some unrelated problem.

Most women are aware of the significance of a lump in the breast and naturally suspect that a nodule in the thyroid could also mean cancer. For this reason, your doctor will probably want you to see a specialist. In fact, the great majority of single thyroid nodules are not cancers of the thyroid.

HOW IS IT DIAGNOSED?

If you have a single thyroid nodule, your blood tests will usually show normal levels of the thyroid hormones T3 and T4 and thyroid-stimulating hormone (TSH). You will be classified medically as "euthyroid." The exception is the toxic adenoma, in which the thyroid blood tests demonstrate an overactive thyroid gland. The thyroid specialist will examine your neck carefully. About half of all patients thought to have a single nodule have, in fact, generalized nodular enlargement of the thyroid known as multinodular goiter. In this case, you can be assured that your condition is unlikely to be serious.

People who need further investigation may have an ultrasound or a radioisotope scan of their thyroid gland. However, the single most important test is fine needle aspiration (FNA) of the nodule (see p.49). The technique is simple, quick, and if necessary can be carried out two or three times because it does not cause significant pain or discomfort. FNA is one of the most important advances in the care of people with thyroid disease. In the past, the majority of patients with a single thyroid nodule had to have surgery, but many operations can now be avoided simply by examining a small sample of thyroid cells obtained by aspiration in the outpatient department. The outcome of the FNA will be one of those indicated in the box below.

Benign or noncancerous nodules may continue to enlarge over many years and eventually get so big that an operation is needed to remove them for the sake of your appearance alone. If you are worried that the nodule is harboring a cancer, your specialist may suggest operating to remove the nodule so that it can be examined microscopically and the question can be resolved once and for all.

What Does Fine Needle Aspiration Reveal?

Fine needle aspiration, in which a few thyroid cells are removed for examination, is used to investigate thyroid nodules. The outcome will be one of the following:

- The needle will remove fluid and the nodule will disappear. This means that the nodule must have been a thyroid cyst, and no further treatment is needed. If the cyst recurs, it can be aspirated again. However, for repeat recurrence, you may need an operation to remove that half of the thyroid gland containing the cyst.
- The cells removed from the nodule show that it is benign and not cancerous. Unless the swelling is sufficiently large to be disfiguring and necessitates surgery, you can be reassured that no treatment is needed.
- The cells removed are malignant, which means that the nodule is thyroid cancer. You will need an operation.
- Sometimes, because of the small number of cells removed, it may be impossible to be certain whether the nodule is benign or malignant. You will then need an operation to remove the entire nodule so that it can be examined carefully under the microscope.

KEY POINTS

- In noniodine-deficient countries, the cause of a goiter is usually unknown.
- Young people with a simple diffuse goiter rarely need any treatment.
- You may be referred to a specialist to have a multinodular goiter investigated and may have several tests.
- A small goiter may be left alone, but you will need regular blood tests done by a doctor because there is a chance of developing hyperthyroidism later.
- An operation or treatment with radioactive iodine may be necessary if a goiter is causing problems.
- Levothyroxine pills may not shrink a goiter; however, they are still prescribed in some countries.
- People who develop thyroid nodules often worry that the lump may be cancer, but this rarely turns out to be the case.
- As a result of the simple and painless investigation known as fine needle aspiration, far fewer people now require surgery.
- If you are concerned about your appearance or cannot stop worrying about the possibility of cancer, you can have an operation to remove the nodule.

Thyroid cancer

Malignant tumors of the thyroid gland are rare. For example, a specialist may see anywhere from 50 to 100 patients with hyperthyroidism caused by Graves' disease for every one patient with thyroid cancer.

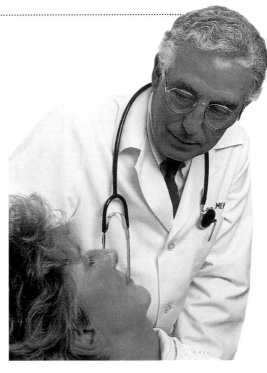

The two types of thyroid cancer that doctors see most often are:
- Papillary cancer, which mostly affects young women and children.
- Follicular cancer, which is unusual before the age of 30.

These two medical terms describe the appearance of the tumor under the microscope. In papillary cancer, the tumor contains papillae or fronds. In follicular cancer, although the appearance is distinctly abnormal, there are still structures that resemble the normal follicles of the thyroid gland. Both types of thyroid cancer can occur at any age. If diagnosis and treatment are carried out at an early stage, the person may have a normal life span. In other words, it is more likely that you will die of a stroke or a heart attack in old age than of thyroid cancer.

CONFIRMING THE DIAGNOSIS
Your doctor will examine any lumps in your neck, but diagnosis of thyroid cancer can be made only after fine needle aspiration or surgery.

HOW IS IT DIAGNOSED?

Most patients visit their doctor with a lump in the neck or because of rapid new growth of a goiter that they have had for many years. The diagnosis of thyroid cancer is usually made by fine needle aspiration or following surgery.

Occasionally, the patient consults his or her doctor because of enlarged lymph nodes in the neck that may at first be thought to be caused by Hodgkin's disease. However, a biopsy will show that the patient actually has papillary cancer that has spread from the thyroid gland through the lymphatic system to the nearby lymph nodes.

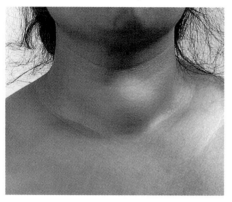

CANCER OF THE THYROID
The first sign of thyroid cancer is a painless nodule in the neck, in or near the thyroid gland.

WHAT IS THE TREATMENT?

Thyroid cancer is normally treated by complete or partial removal of the thyroid gland. Radioactive iodine is commonly used after the operation to kill any remaining cancerous cells.

SURGERY

Papillary cancer is usually treated by removing as much of the thyroid gland as possible. A total thyroidectomy is performed because the cancer may occur in various places throughout the gland. Any large lymph nodes containing the cancer are also removed at this stage. In contrast, follicular cancer usually develops in only one part of the thyroid and removal of half of the gland, known as hemi-thyroidectomy, may be all that is necessary.

No special treatment is required before the operation and you can usually go home after two or three days.

RADIOACTIVE IODINE

It is not possible to remove every last part of the thyroid gland by means of surgery. Some patients who have been diagnosed with papillary cancer will be given a large dose of radioactive iodine (iodine-131) to kill any remaining cells. The radioactive iodine is given as a liquid or a capsule in the hospital. You will then have to stay in the hospital for 24–48 hours and you will be separated from other patients and their visitors in a single room in order to avoid contaminating them with radioactivity.

The radioactive iodine is usually administered four weeks after your operation and before treatment with levothyroxine pills has been started. The iodine is most effective when the patient is hypothyroid and the blood level of thyroid-stimulating hormone (TSH) is high. If for some reason you have already started taking levothyroxine to prevent you from becoming hypothyroid after removal of your thyroid gland, you will be taken off the treatment about four weeks before being given radioactive iodine. Toward the end of the period without levothyroxine, you may feel tired.

LEVOTHYROXINE

Doctors believe that the rate of growth of papillary and follicular cancers of the thyroid may be increased by the hormone TSH. It is important to take enough levo-thyroxine to ensure that the level of TSH in your blood becomes undetectable. Patients with thyroid cancer need a slightly greater dose of levothyroxine than those with hypothyroidism. A dose of 150 to 200 micrograms daily is usually enough to switch off TSH secretion by the pituitary gland.

HOW IS IT FOLLOWED?

Like the normal thyroid gland, papillary and follicular cancers make a substance called thyroglobulin. The thyroid gland normally secretes this substance only in the presence of TSH, but this is not the case with thyroid cancer. If there is no TSH detectable in the bloodstream because it has been suppressed by treatment with levothyroxine, any thyroglobulin in the blood must be coming from recurrent cancer in the neck or from cancer that has spread to other parts of the body, known as secondary cancer or metastases. Thyroglobulin is therefore known as a "tumor marker." If a patient who is taking appropriate amounts of levothyroxine has an elevated level of thyroglobulin, the specialist may wish to perform a scan of the whole body using radioactive iodine to identify the site of the recurrent tumor or its metastases.

FINDING A TUMOR
An isotope scan can identify the site of a recurrent tumor or its metastases. Cancerous cells are seen on this scan as white and yellow areas in the patient's neck.

The scan is usually performed 24–48 hours after a dose of iodine-131 by mouth, four weeks after the patient has stopped taking levothyroxine or after TSH injections. Recently, it has become possible to increase the level of TSH in the blood by giving injections of synthetic TSH (thyrogen), which is identical to that made by the human pituitary gland, and thereby avoid the need to stop levothyroxine treatment. Any tumor that is found may be treated with a large dose of radioactive iodine.

WHAT IS THE OUTLOOK?

The outlook depends upon the size of the tumor and whether it has spread at the time of diagnosis. If treated correctly, a young woman with a small papillary cancer of the thyroid is likely to have a normal life expectancy, even if the cancer has spread to the lymph nodes in the neck. Even patients with follicular cancer that has spread to the bones or lungs may survive for many years with a good quality of life.

Case History: **ENLARGED LYMPH NODES**

Susan Jones was 18 when she fell heavily, striking the side of her neck. As the pain and bruising improved she noticed a pea-sized lump in her neck. At first, her doctor thought that the lump was related to the accident. However, the lump moved when she swallowed, suggesting that it lay within the thyroid gland.

When the lump had not disappeared after six weeks, the doctor referred Susan to a thyroid specialist. The specialist examined Susan's neck and found a single small thyroid nodule and three enlarged lymph nodes on the right side. He took a tiny sample from the thyroid nodule and one of the lymph nodes, removing cells with a syringe and needle. The test took only a few minutes, requiring no local anesthesia and causing Susan no discomfort.

The next day Susan was informed that the lump in her neck was a type of cancer of the thyroid, known as papillary carcinoma, and that it had spread to the nearby lymph nodes. Two weeks later, Susan was admitted to the hospital, and almost all of her thyroid gland was removed along with the enlarged lymph nodes. Careful inspection of the removed gland by pathologists showed no other signs of thyroid cancer apart from the original swelling.

After followup treatment with radioactive iodine, Susan has been cured and she simply needs to take levothyroxine pills for the rest of her life and see the specialist every year for a blood test.

RARE CANCERS

Rare forms of thyroid cancer include the following:

- Medullary cancer of the thyroid, which can occur on its own or run in families. It may or may not be associated with abnormalities of other endocrine glands or of the skeleton.
- Lymphoma of the thyroid, which usually affects elderly people and may be accompanied by evidence of disease in other parts of the body.
- Anaplastic cancer, which also affects elderly people.

The future prospects for people with these types of cancer is not as good as those with papillary or follicular cancer. Treatment is more difficult and may include chemotherapy and radiation therapy.

KEY POINTS

- Thyroid cancer is rare.
- The two types of cancer that doctors most often see, papillary and follicular, can normally be treated successfully if they are diagnosed early.
- Depending on the type of cancer, an operation is necessary to remove all or part of the thyroid gland. Papillary cancer may require subsequent treatment with radioactive iodine to destroy any remaining cells.
- After treatment of thyroid cancer with surgery and radioactive iodine, levothyroxine is taken for life.
- Blood tests and scans will be done after treatment to be sure that no trace of cancer remains in the body.
- A few very rare cancers that mainly affect elderly people are more difficult to treat.

Thyroid blood tests

Increasingly, patients wish to know about the actual levels of thyroid hormones and thyroid-stimulating hormone (TSH) in the blood. The normal, or reference, ranges for these hormones are shown in the box on page 62.

The normal, or reference, ranges for thyroid hormones T3 and T4 and TSH will vary slightly from laboratory to laboratory, depending upon the normal population used for the calculations and upon the type of assay used for the measurement of the hormones. The thyroid hormones T3 and T4 are almost exclusively bound to a protein in the bloodstream and, as such, are inactive. Less than one percent of these hormones is unbound or free and able to control the metabolism of the body.

Measurement of total T3 and T4 includes both bound and free hormones, whereas measurement of free T4 and T3 excludes the much larger bound hormones. Measurement of free and total thyroid hormones usually provides the same information on whether the thyroid is working normally or in an over- or underactive state. Laboratories usually offer measurement of total thyroid hormones and free thyroid hormones.

LABORATORY TESTS
Tests are available to measure the levels of thyroid hormones and TSH in the blood.

Normal Hormone Reference Ranges

This table shows the normal reference ranges of thyroid hormone and TSH levels in the blood. Your doctor or specialist will compare your blood tests with these figures to assess your condition.

HORMONE	REFERENCE RANGE
Total thyroxine (TT4)	4.5–11.5 ug/dl
Free thyroxine (fT4)	7.5–20 ng/dl
Total triiodothyronine (TT3)	90–180 ng/dl
Free triiodothyronine (fT3)	20–40 pg/dl
Thyrotropin, or thyroid-stimulating hormone (TSH)	0.5–5.0 milliunits per liter (mU/l)

microgram = 10^{-6} gram   nanogram = 10^{-9} gram   picogram = 10^{-12} gram

For the scientifically minded, a mole is the molecular weight of a substance in grams.

- A mole of thyroxine is 777 grams.
- A nanomole of thyroxine is 777 nanograms (or 777×10^{-9} grams)
- A picomole of thyroxine is 777 picograms (or 777×10^{-12} grams).

Most hormones are now measured in molar units, which are believed to reflect activity more accurately. However, drugs are still prescribed in mass units or grams. A dose of 100 micrograms (or 100×10^{-6} grams) of thyroxine is the equivalent of about 130 nanomoles.

TYPICAL RESULTS

Generally speaking, the more severe the symptoms of over- or underactivity of the thyroid gland, the more abnormal the results of the thyroid blood tests. However, in older patients in whom hyperthyroidism may be no less serious and who have heart complications such as an irregular heartbeat caused by atrial fibrillation, the levels of thyroid hormones T3 and T4 may be only marginally elevated.

With very rare exceptions, the TSH level in the blood of patients with hyperthyroidism is so low that it cannot be detected.

By the time that patients with hypothyroidism develop typical symptoms, fT4 and TT4 levels are low and associated with an elevated TSH level in the blood. However, with increased patient screening, more patients without symptoms are found to have hypothyroidism. Rarely, hypothyroidism is the result of disease of the pituitary gland and not of the thyroid gland. In such cases, low fT4 or TT4 is combined with a normal or low level of TSH.

In mild or subclinical hypothyroidism (see p.36), fT4 and TT4 lie in the lower part of the normal range and are usually associated with a TSH level in the blood of between 5 and 10 mU/l.

Blood levels of T3 may be used to evaluate those patients who have hyperthyroidism, but they are not routinely measured in patients who are suspected of having hypothyroidism.

DETERMINING THE CORRECT DOSE OF LEVOTHYROXINE

Your primary care physician or thyroid specialist will usually prescribe a dose of levothyroxine that raises the fT4 and TT4 to within the normal range and reduces the TSH level in the blood to the lower part of the normal range. In some patients, a sense of well-being is achieved only when fT4 or TT4 is raised and TSH is low or undetectable. In this circumstance, it is essential that the T3 level in the blood be maintained in the normal range in order to avoid hyperthyroidism.

If you are not taking your levothyroxine regularly, it will be obvious from the blood test results.

— EFFECT OF ILLNESS ON THYROID —

Illness, whether sudden, such as pneumonia or a heart attack, or of long duration, such as rheumatoid arthritis or depression, may affect the results of thyroid blood tests and give the impression of hyper- or hypothyroidism. This is known as the "euthyroid-sick" syndrome. It is possible that, after referral to a specialist and further investigation, no underlying thyroid disease will be found.

Warning

Thyroid blood tests should not be interpreted in isolation. Appropriate medical care will also depend on careful assessment of symptoms and clinical examination.

KEY POINTS

- Different laboratories use slightly different normal ranges.
- In most cases, the more severe the symptoms of thyroid malfunction, the more abnormal blood test results will be.
- Blood test results enable the specialist or primary care physician to determine the necessary dose of levothyroxine.
- Some other illnesses can produce thyroid blood test results that falsely suggest hyper- or hypothyroidism.

Questions and answers

Does diet affect my thyroid and its function?

You may have heard that iodine has something to do with the thyroid gland. Indeed, iodine is an integral part of the thyroxine (T4) and triiodothyronine (T3) molecules produced by the thyroid gland. A lack of iodine in the diet may cause a goiter or even hypothyroidism. This is commonly found in people who live in mountainous areas far from the sea, such as the Himalayas. However, the diet in the US contains adequate amounts of iodine. You do not need to take supplements. For the nonbelievers, iodized salt is available in some supermarkets. Excessive iodine intake, however, may unmask underlying thyroid disease and produce either hyperthyroidism or hypothyroidism.

Is smoking harmful?

The eye disease that accompanies Graves' disease is more common and more severe among patients who smoke. Patients with hyperthyroidism caused by Graves' disease should stop smoking.

Was stress responsible for making my thyroid gland overactive?

Although it is difficult to prove, most thyroid specialists are impressed by how often major life events, such as divorce or death of a close relative, appear to have taken place a few months before the onset of hyperthyroidism caused by Graves' disease. There is now evidence that stress can affect the immune system, which is abnormal in Graves' disease. So the answer may be "yes," but there are other important factors, such as heredity.

Will my new baby have thyroid trouble?

The children of a mother who has Graves' disease or a previous history of Graves' disease may be born with an overactive thyroid gland. This is known as neonatal thyrotoxicosis and lasts for only a few weeks. The obstetrician and the pediatrician will look out for this rare complication, which is readily treated. Occasionally, mothers who have hypothyroidism give birth to a child with an underactive thyroid gland. Again, this condition is usually short-lived and will be detected by the routine blood testing of all babies a few days after birth.

Will my children be affected by autoimmune thyroid disease if I have it?

Not necessarily. In fact, the risk is relatively small, although it is greater than that for children who have no family history of autoimmune disease. Nor is it always the same autoimmune disease that runs in families. For example, a mother may have Graves' disease, while her daughter may develop insulin-dependent diabetes mellitus.

Could my thyroid condition explain why I did badly in my college entrance exams?

It is likely to be hyperthyroidism that affects people at the high-school age. If not adequately treated, hyperthyroidism can result in a reduced ability to concentrate and lead to a substandard performance.

Could thyroid disease have caused my anxiety/depression?

The answer is usually "no," but in some patients, anxiety or depression are entirely attributed to thyroid disease. Hyperthyroidism and hypothyroidism will almost always make underlying psychiatric illness worse. Unfortunately, even when a person who suffers from hyperthyroidism is successfully treated and the overactive thyroid is brought under control, the psychiatric symptoms do not disappear altogether, although they may improve.

Will my Graves' disease recur?

If your hyperthyroidism has been effectively treated with iodine-131, the condition will rarely return. If the hyperthyroidism has resolved after a single course of methimazole, there is a 30–50 percent chance of recurrence, usually within one to two years of stopping the drug. Recurrent hyperthyroidism after surgery is usually apparent within a few weeks but may occur as long as 40 years after apparently successful surgery.

Does it matter if I forget to take my medication?

The occasional missed pill is not the end of the world. Since symptoms of hypothyroidism caused by lack of levothyroxine are not usually felt for two to three weeks after stopping the treatment, it would still be possible to enjoy a 7–10-day vacation if you inadvertently left your medication at home. However, this is not recommended. Also, patients with hypothyroidism may have other autoimmune diseases, such as diabetes mellitus. Failure to take levothyroxine regularly will affect the response to insulin and may lead to unexpected coma as a result of low blood sugar.

Likewise, missing the odd dose of methimazole will not cause significant problems, but symptoms of hyperthyroidism can develop if you don't take the pills for 24–48 hours, especially within a few weeks of starting treatment.

I feel better when I am taking a higher dose of levothyroxine than prescribed by my doctor. Is this safe?
There is considerable debate about the correct dose of levothyroxine. The consensus is that enough should be given to ensure that blood levels of T4 are within the limits of normal or slightly elevated, and of TSH at the lower limit of normal or, in some patients, lower.

By taking excessive levothyroxine, a sense of well-being, increased energy, and even weight loss may be achieved in the short term. However, there are long-term dangers to the heart and a possibility of increasing the rate of bone thinning and therefore encouraging the development of osteoporosis. You should never change your levothyroxine dose without discussing it with your physician.

Glossary

This glossary explains the meaning of the most frequently used terms connected with the diagnosis and treatment of thyroid disorders.

antibodies: proteins produced by the body's immune system as a defense mechanism against "foreign" protein contained, for example, in bacteria. Antibodies are not normally formed against proteins that are part of the body but do occur in people with autoimmune disease.

autoimmune disease: inappropriate production of antibodies that are directed against parts of the body. For example, in most patients with hypothyroidism, antibodies are formed that participate in the destruction of the thyroid gland. In Graves' disease, antibodies directed against the surface of the thyroid cell stimulate overproduction of thyroid hormones.

de Quervain's thyroiditis: a form of thyroiditis that can occur following a viral infection of the thyroid.

exophthalmos: prominence of the eyes most commonly found in patients with hyperthyroidism caused by Graves' disease. Exophthalmos may affect one or both eyes, may be apparent before the overactive thyroid gland develops, and may appear for the first time after successful treatment of the hyperthyroidism.

fine needle aspiration (FNA): a test that involves passing a small needle into the thyroid gland and sucking out or aspirating a small sample of tissue for examination under the microscope. This technique often avoids the need for surgery in patients who have a thyroid nodule.

goiter: an enlarged thyroid gland.

Graves' disease: the name given to the most common form of hyperthyroidism. Patients often have exophthalmos, a goiter, and sometimes raised red patches on the legs, known as pretibial myxedema.

Hashimoto's thyroiditis: the name given to a particular kind of goiter caused by autoimmune disease. Although the thyroid gland is enlarged, there is often evidence of hypothyroidism.

hyperthyroidism: the condition resulting from an overactive thyroid gland.

hypothyroidism: the condition resulting from an underactive thyroid gland.

methimazole: the drug most commonly used in the US in the treatment of hyperthyroidism. It acts by interfering with excessive production of thyroid hormones.

myxedema: a term for hypothyroidism that is often used to describe patients in whom the underactivity of the thyroid gland is severe and long-standing.

postpartum thyroiditis: a transient disturbance in the balance of the thyroid gland that can occur in the first year after childbirth. There are usually no symptoms, but there may be symptoms of hyperthyroidism or of hypothyroidism. Treatment is usually not necessary.

propranolol: a drug belonging to the group known as beta blockers, which alleviate some of the symptoms in patients with an overactive thyroid gland. Other members of the group include nadolol and metoprolol.

proptosis: another word for exophthalmos.

propylthiouracil: a drug with a similar action to methimazole. It is used if patients develop side effects to methimazole or for hyperthyroidism in patients who are breast-feeding.

radioactive iodine: isotopes of iodine used in the investigation and treatment of hyperthyroidism. Iodine-123 is used for most scans; iodine-131 is used for treatment.

tetany: a condition that results from a low level of calcium in the blood and is characterized by tingling in the hands, feet, and around the mouth and by painful spasm of the muscles of the hands and feet.

thyroglobulin: a protein secreted by the thyroid gland. Its measurement is an important part of the follow-up of patients who have been treated for thyroid cancer. It is known as a "tumor marker" because its presence in certain situations may indicate that the cancer has recurred in other parts of the body.

thyrotoxicosis: another term for hyperthyroidism.

thyrotropin (thyroid-stimulating hormone or TSH): a hormone secreted by the pituitary gland that is responsible for controlling the output of thyroid hormones by the thyroid gland. In hypothyroidism caused by disease of the thyroid gland, TSH concentrations are elevated in the blood, and in hyperthyroidism TSH concentrations are low.

thyroxine (T4): one of the two hormones that are secreted by the thyroid gland. It has to be converted in the body to triiodothyronine before it is active. Thyroxine is available in pill form as levothyroxine, a synthetic thyroxine, for the treatment of hypothyroidism.

triiodothyronine (T3): one of the two hormones that are secreted by the thyroid gland and are responsible for controlling the metabolism of the body. Although available in pill form, it is not usually prescribed for patients with hypothyroidism because it does not provide as good control as thyroxine.

Useful addresses

The Thyroid Center
Online: cpmcnet.columbia.edu/dept/ thyroid
Columbia-Presbyterian Center
161 Fort Washington Avenue
New York, NY 10032
Tel: (212) 305-0440

American Thyroid Association
Online: www.thyroid.org
Montefiore Medical Center
111 East 210th Street
Bronx, NY 10467
Tel: (718) 882-6085

The Thyroid Foundation of America
Online: www.tsh.org
Ruth Sleeper Hall
40 Parkman Street
Boston, MA 02114-2698
Tel: (800) 832-8321

The Thyroid Society
Online: www.the-thyroid-society.org
7515 South Main Street
Houston, TX 77030
Tel: (800) THYROID

Index

Acknowledgments

PUBLISHER'S ACKNOWLEDGMENTS
Dorling Kindersley Publishing, Inc. would like to thank the following for their help
and participation in this project:

Managing Editor Stephanie Jackson; **Managing Art Editor** Nigel Duffield;
Editorial Assistance Mary Lindsay, Ann Mummery, Jennifer Quasha, Ashley Ren,
Design Revolution; **Design Assistance** Sarah Hall, Design Revolution, Chris Walker;
Production Michelle Thomas, Elizabeth Cherry;
Consultancy Dr. Tony Smith, Dr. Sue Davidson;
Indexing Indexing Specialists, Hove; **Administration** Christopher Gordon.

Illustrations (p.8) ©Philip Wilson; (p.9) Neal Johnson;
Picture Research Angela Anderson; **Picture Librarian** Charlotte Oster.

PICTURE CREDITS
The publisher would like to thank the following for their kind permission to reproduce
their photographs. Every effort has been made to trace the copyright holders. Dorling Kindersley
apologizes for any unintentional omissions and would be pleased, in any such cases, to add
an acknowledgment in future editions.

National Medical Slide Bank p.10, p.56; **Science Photo Library** p.7 (John Burbidge),
p.26 (Dr. P. Marazzi), p.42 (Ron Sutherland), p.55 (John Greim),
p.58 (Oulette Theroux), p.61 (Sinclair Stammers).